Resetting your adrenals

A guide to detoxing and getting back on track

Contents

Feeling "Off"?

Did you know your adrenal glands produce over 50 different hormones? When they are not working correctly, you can have mood swings, fatigue, and other symptoms related to having adrenals that are full of toxins, causing them not to function properly. This book walks you through how to get them back to peak performance.

Introduction

Your adrenals work harder than you think. They regulate at least 50 different types of hormones which regulate everything from sex drive to weight loss. This book will teach you:

What are adrenal glands and what are their functions.
The symptoms of adrenal stress or fatigue
.How to detoxify your adrenals
What foods to avoid making the adrenals work properly.
What exercises are recommended for peaks and valleys

Chapter 1: Your adrenals and you

Your adrenal glands are located on top of your kidneys. Their very name means above (ad) kidneys (renal). It is important to know where they are and what they do in regards your body so you have an idea of when they are not functioning as they should.

They are no bigger than a walnut, but they regulate over 50 different hormones, including estrogen, testosterone, adrenaline, cortisol, and other steroids, among others. They sit, like a pyramid and weigh no more than a grape.

When your body is under stress or during physical activity, they release the appropriate amount of the corresponding hormone to regulate your breathing, energy, and flight-or-fight responses.

They help back up the pancreas, helping regulate blood sugar, and help your immune system in times of high stress. During puberty, and throughout life, they help the female and male reproductive systems maintain the correct levels of hormones to aid in sex drive, and procreation.

When you maintain a proper diet and low stress lifestyle, your adrenals work normally, regulating all the functions they need to in order for you to remain in good health. However, when the wrong foods, sedentary lifestyle, and constantly stressful situations persist, they become bogged down and try to work overtime, leading to a condition called adrenal fatigue.

This syndrome causes over-all fatigue in the body. Some of the symptoms include:

Feeling tired after having a normal sleep period.
Running out of energy or being easily overwhelmed in stressful situations or doing everyday routines.
Not recovering from illness as you once,
Having a constant need to eat salty or sweet foods.

Your energy levels are higher in the evening than when you first wake up.

All these can be signs of adrenal fatigue and they must be addressed by going to a licensed physician. Ignoring these signs can lead to more serious illnesses later in life.

Do I have adrenal fatigue?

Though it is generally recommended that you see a physician to properly diagnose adrenal fatigue, there are ways you can test for it at home before you tell your doctor of your concerns:

Horizontal Blood pressure check

Lie on your back perfectly still and relax for five minutes. Take your blood pressure while lying down. After taking it lying down, stand up and take it again. Under normal circumstances, your blood pressure should rise between 10-20 points. If it drops ten or more, your adrenals may not be functioning properly.

Check your irises

The iris is the black part of your eyes that regulates the amount of light you need to see. With a flashlight or similar light source, stand in a pitch dark room, allowing your irises to dilate, or become enlarged. After they have adjusted to the darkness, turn on the light source and look in the mirror. If they contract and stay contracted, they are normal. If they fluctuate between being contracted and trying to relax to take in lighter, you need to have your adrenals checked.

The White Line test

With an edge of a spoon or fingernail, draw a line across your belly, if it turns red, this is normal. If it remains white or stays white and enlarges, it may be a sign of a serious adrenal problem and needs to be addressed with your doctor.

Once you schedule an appointment with your physician, let him/her know all the symptoms you are suffering from as well as the home tests that you have performed on yourself. Let him/her also know what supplements you are currently taking and any dietary changes you have done before arriving at the office. Do not withhold any information.

To make it easier on your doctor, it is best to keep a record of how you have been feeling, your diet, and any medications and supplements you are taking. This will help your doctor work with you on a solution, and a course of action you need to take to reset your adrenals.

Chapter 2: What you can't eat...

Once you are diagnosed with an adrenal condition, your next step is getting on the path to cleansing and resetting them back to normal levels. There are many diets out there that do this, but we are going to walk your through an easy way to get started on the path to health.

This means taking everything you know about a regular diet and throwing it out the window.

Don't eat "diet" food

These are foods that are fat free, or low on carbohydrates. Many of these foods are highly processed and will actually do more harm than good when you're on the road to recovery.

Avoid refined sugars and flours.

Any food that is highly refined will convert immediately into sugar leading to a spike in your sugar and throwing your body into a sugar spiral where you will need to consume more sugar to keep your energy going. This is detrimental to your health for more than just your adrenals.

Any foods that have been enriched fall into this category as well. Enriched foods have had their natural nutrients stripped from them and replaced during the enrichment process.

Avoid Sports drinks, energy drinks and caffeinated beverages.

Sports drinks contain high fructose corn syrup, which is a refined sugar. I will have a recipe for an electrolyte drink you can make yourself in a later chapter. Energy drinks and drinks with caffeine will make your body dependent on them for the energy they give you, making you crave more and more caffeine, which will tax your adrenals even further.

Weaning off of Caffeine

If you are already a drinker of energy drinks or other caffeinated beverages, weaning yourself off them is best. Start by eliminating one can or cup at a time, allowing your body to adjust to the new intake until you can go completely without them. Your energy levels will return to normal, and your adrenal glands will thank you.

Avoid alcoholic beverages.

Alcohol depletes the system of the vitamins and minerals your adrenals need to function at normal levels, causing to fatigue at a rapid rate. Cutting alcohol out completely is recommended.

Weaning off of alcohol

If you frequently consume a substantial amount of alcohol, abruptly stopping may result in complications. It is recommended that you gradually wean yourself off of alcoholic beverages. Your physician can help you in this regard. Going cold turkey can lead to rapid detox, giving you the shakes and other harsh withdrawal symptoms that will further tax your adrenals.

Limit sour fruits and fruits and vegetables that are high in natural sugars.

Bananas are high on this list because they have high potassium levels that can throw off adrenal glands during this process. Choose non-starchy fruits and vegetables. If you like your broccoli, cabbage and greens, cook them fully before eating them to reduce the thyroid inhibiting enzyme they naturally have.

Fruits with high sugar content include bananas, figs, grapes, guava, kumquat, lychee, mango, persimmon, and pomegranate.

Vegetables that are high in sugar include all potatoes, beets, carrots, corn, parsnips, peas, plantains, and winter squashes, (especially acorn and butternut).

Pay attention to your body's signals regarding salt intake.

If your body is craving salt, make it Sea Salt. Sea Salt has all the vitamins and minerals that iodized salt does not, making it the better choice for salt when on the road to adrenal recovery.

Pinpoint and avoid allergens

Your doctor can help you with identifying food and other allergens. Avoiding these can help not only your adrenals, but your body as a whole. By avoiding foods that cause allergic reactions, you're reducing system stresses that can tax your adrenals and your immune system.

Chapter 3: What you can eat

Just when you begin to think that you will be reduced to lettuce and other vegetables, here is a list of foods that you can eat to reset your adrenals and insure a long and healthy life.

Rethink your breakfast foods.

Instead of grabbing a shake or pre-mixed smoothie, or even fixing yourself a bowl of cereal, reach for breakfast foods high in protein. Eggs, bacon, and sausage are three that come to mind immediately.

If you want your smoothie in the morning, use nuts for your protein, preferably raw nuts that have been soaked overnight. Use also unsweetened nut milks and plain yogurt. If you want a little sweet, raw honey, Grade B Maple Syrup, and Stevia are your best bets.

Go whole and organic foods

The closer your food is to its natural state, the better it will be for you and your adrenals. Whole Wheat, millet, and other whole grains for bread and crackers and no chips. Organic foods are also a boost to adrenal health as they do not contain the toxins from pesticides and genetically modified foods.

Do not avoid fats, just eat the right ones.

Your body needs cholesterol and fat to produce hormones. Organic butter from grass fed cows, olive oil for salad dressings, and use coconut oil and Grapeseed oil for sautéing and frying are all good options. The latter two can stand up to high heat for baking and frying.

Eat Real food

Do not buy pre-made box meals. They contain enzymes and chemicals that tax your system and can set your road to health back a few steps. Buy fresh foods. Use the alternative noodles to cook. These include buckwheat noodles, whole wheat noodles and noodles made with vegetables. It may take some getting used to eating, but your body will thank you in the long run.

If you must eat out,

Tell the server you don't want them to brush your food with margarine. This is a trick they employ to make the meats juicier. They do have actual butter. Ask for that instead. Avoid anything fried in restaurants. They cook foods in vegetable oils that can be detrimental. Ask for the dressings on the side and dip your salad in the dressing.

Choose high protein foods and skip the rolls. We all like rolls, but they are pre-made with refined flours that can throw your adrenals into a fit. Avoid any noodle dishes as they contain enriched processed noodles.

Chapter 4: Supplements to get you back on track

There are a lot of combinations of supplements out there for resetting your adrenals, but some may contain ingredients to which you may be allergic or may react to medications you are already taking.

This is a list of vitamins and herbals that you can take to your doctor so the both of you can decide on the right ones for you. This is only a guideline and everybody metabolizes nutrients and herbals at different rates.

Vitamins and Minerals

Magnesium is on the top of the list when it comes to relieving stress and coming back to a normal sleep rhythm. There is a fine balance to taking magnesium and it must be done at small doses at the start. There are places online that you can buy magnesium powder. This can be mixed in water.

Vitamin C is vital for proper adrenal health. This vitamin helps to rebuild tissue and to help the adrenals get back to normal. Vitamin C aids in the production of norepinephrine, epinephrine, dopamine, and helps in the making of testosterone, cortisol, and aldosterone. The minimal dose should be 1500mg a day.

Balanced B Vitamins are also good for helping to manage stress. By taking a balanced combination of these vitamins, it will help your body better handle highly stressful situations and provide you with natural energy and mental focus, which often tends to wane when your body is taxed. For more severe cases, buy B5 as an added supplement to your B vitamins.

Zinc is an immune booster, but it can help manage stress and help your adrenals reset faster. It is also a natural energy booster. Your doctor needs to set your dosage.

Cortisol supplements are out there to help with this condition, but I highly recommended taking it under doctors' orders as this can be abused leading to other problems.

Herbal Supplements

When looking at resetting adrenals using herbals, we have to look at them separately and start with adaptogens. These kinds of herbs assess your body's needs and strengthen the weaknesses they find.

Ashwaghanda Root (Withania somnifera) is an herb of the nightshade family that is a very potent adaptogen. If your body is low on hormones, this herb will produce the ones of which you are in need. It's also an energy booster, and helps the body fight against the effects of stress and anxiety.

Astragalus Root (Astragali membranaceus) is another adaptogen that helps to regulate body functions. It helps to boost the immune system and helps to combat fatigue brought on by stressful situations. It also aids in fighting the chronic fatigue that accompanies adrenal fatigue.

Siberian Ginseng (Eleutherococcus senticosus) has been used for centuries in herbalism. This adaptogen helps to normalize response of the immune system, aids in bringing hormones back into balance, and increases endurance. In doing all of these, it takes the stress off of the adrenals, helping to bring them back to normal function as well.

Balancing your hormones naturally is also a key to resetting your adrenals and getting back to a healthy life. Here is a list of herbals that you can take in a combination to help restore your hormone levels.

For the Ladies

Wild Yam (Dioscorea villosa) is an herb that contains a precursor to progesterone. It helps the body produce this cancer fighting hormone and will also help bring the adrenals back to healthy functions. This usually comes in a cream and must be used as directed.

Black Cohosh (Cimifuga recemosa) is a well-known herb in menopausal circles as it can bring the estrogen in the body back into balance. In so doing, it also takes the stress off of the adrenals. This will allow the glands to reset without complications.

Damiana (Turnera aphrodisiaca) Is a long standing herb that is often taken in conjunction with Black Cohosh to regulate the hormones. It also helps to combat fatigue.

For the Men

Saw Palmetto (Serenoa repens) is an herb that has been used by Native Americans for blood pressure regulation and glandular problems. It helps to bring male hormones back into balance and to reinforce and strengthen the glandular system as a whole, making this herb key in resetting adrenals not only in men, but woman as well.

Sarsaparilla (Smilax ornata) is a root that is often used with Saw Palmetto for regulating hormones and the glandular system in men. It acts much like the above herb in helping to reset the adrenal glands and bring them back to health.

For Both

A key problem in adrenal malfunction is the inability to regulate blood sugar, which may worsen diabetes and hypoglycemia. Here are a few herbs that can help in that area.

Nopal (Opuntia ficus-indica) otherwise known as prickly pear, is a forerunner in the regulation of blood sugar. It help the body produce the insulin necessary to regulate sugars in the blood, taking much of the stress of off the adrenals. There are extracts and capsules on the market, but eating the organic fresh fruit are best.

Stevia (Stevia rebaudiana) is an herbal sweetener that regulates blood sugar and also helps to curve food cravings that are often associated with detox and reset diets. The best form to use this herb is in extract form. You may be able to find a pure granulated form in health food stores.

There is one herbal that comes highly recommended in resetting adrenals.

Juniper Berries (Juniperus species) are well-known to help regulate and rest any adrenal complications. They nutritionally feed and strengthen the adrenal glands, helping them to reset faster; therefore, bringing them back to functioning normally. It also has the added benefit of regulating blood sugar as well. The berries can be juiced and the juice itself can be diluted with water and taken as a beverage.

Herbals for stress

Lavender Flowers (Lavandula angustifolia) are well known for calming nerves and reducing stress. It can be made into a tea or the essential oil can be placed in a diffuser for the same effect. It can also be mixed with other herbs for tea as well.

Green Tea (decaf) is has many beneficial compounds to help cope with and relieve stress. It also has antioxidants which help to give the immune system a boost.

Chamomile Flowers (anthemis Nobilis) mixed with the Lavender above will provide the perfect tea blend when it comes to relaxing and relieving stress. It will also help calm you so you can sleep.

Chapter 5: Managing the peaks and valleys of stress

During the reset, you may experience high and low levels of cortisol. This will cause your energy levels to peak and valley, because your body is trying to manage stresses. Here are a few ways to help your body out.

Meditation/Breathing exercises

Meditation isn't only for gurus and martial artists. The only thing it takes to meditate is to focus on one point or action. Here are a few things you can try:

Close your eyes, and focus on your breath. Breathe in through your nose, slowly, counting seconds as you inhale. Now, put your lips together as if to whistle, and slowly exhale, counting as you did when you inhaled. This is called breathing meditation.

As you breathe in, tense up a muscle group. Hold the tension until you begin to exhale. Relax the muscle group. So this with each group. This is a relaxation exercise that can help you sleep.

Deep breathing is much like the breathing exercise above, but you only do the exercise once or twice, until you can feel the stress leave your body. Just remember not to breathe in or out too fast. It needs to be done slowly for the most effect.

Low energy days

Low energy days are days when your cortisol level is very low, making a restful sleep impossible and leaving you with no or low energy. You still need to move, but you just can't bring yourself to jog, or do a full high-energy workout.

Yoga has many simple and easy routines. One of these routines is the sun salutation:

Because of its slow and purposeful movements, this series of stretches is perfect for a low energy day. If you are not that flexible, bend as far as you can. It's not about flexibility; it's about resetting your adrenals to get you back to feeling like yourself. Do this series about four times.

Lie flat on your back and rest your legs at a ninety degree angle against the wall and breathe. This will stimulate blood flow to the kidneys and adrenals.

Taking a slow stroll can also be beneficial. Not too fast, just regular paced to get the body moving and the blood pumping.

Thai Chi and Qi Gong are two more exercise routines that are perfect for low energy days.

During these times, taking American Ginseng and drinking Chamomile tea will also help. For concentration and mental fatigue that can happen on these days add either Ginkgo Biloba or Gotu kola, both help with memory retention and focus.

For boosts of energy during the day, try eating a serving of nuts. They will not only give you energy, but they contain the protein your body needs to help the adrenals.

Vitamin B12 will also help on these days.

High Stress Days

These are the days you feel wired all the time. You can't seem to calm down, and everything gets on your nerves. You feel like a ticking time bomb.

These days are perfect for weight training and high intensity exercises to burn off the extra stress. Kick-boxing, jogging, anything that keeps you moving for twenty minutes to an hour is perfect. It gets your mind of the stress and you're getting exercise that helps your heart and your adrenals by burning not only fat, but excess energy and stress.

For women, primrose before bedtime will help to further manage the stress so you can sleep.

For everyone, a tea with lemon balm and lavender will soothe nerves and melt stress, leaving you relaxed and ready sleep. You can also use essential oils like geranium and chamomile for high stress days. Put five drops of each in a diffuser and plug it into a socket.

Fluctuating levels

These days make you feel like you are on an energy roller coaster. You're tired in the morning, all over the map during the day, and you feel like running a marathon before bed, causing insomnia.

This is when adaptogenic herbs, like ashwagandha really shine by synthesizing the enzymes needed to even out the energy levels. A combination of ashwagandha, Siberian ginseng, and Stevia will help to bring your levels back into balance. Made into a strong tea will make it more effective.

Eat energy and protein foods in the morning, like nuts and greens. In the evening, break out the meats and make them with brown rice, and green beans. It will leave you feeling full you and your energy levels where they should be for the evening. If you are still too wired to sleep, mix lavender and chamomile with peppermint as a tea for the evening.

Cardio exercises of varying intensity throughout the day will help to level out the fluctuating cortisol and energy levels. When they are low, do a little yoga or go for a short leisurely walk. If they are high, try aerobic exercises or a treadmill or stair stepper.

Chapter 6: Making alternatives...

We all love our respective drinks, and often can't fathom life without ingesting them, but when you're trying to reset your adrenals, you have to make the sacrifices. When it comes to some of your favorite food and drinks, you can make alternatives that taste just a good without all the sugars and caffeine that comes with them.

Hold the Coffee

Before reaching for that coffee, go for the chicory instead. To even out its full-bodied taste, it can be tempered with a little cinnamon and orange peel. Place one tablespoon of chicory per six ounce cup of water.

When you're finished adding the chicory, place either 1/8 teaspoon of either the orange zest or cinnamon in the grinds before brewing. If you want to sweeten it, use raw honey or stevia.

Pass the energy drinks and sports drinks...

Making or buying unsweetened nut milks will give you the best boost of energy. If you must have an energy drink, try this:

1/2 cup of Strawberries or Raspberries juiced
20 ounces of coconut water
1/4 tsp sea salt
1/2 tsp of Unsulfured Black Strap molasses

Blend all of them together in a blender and enjoy. This electrolyte packed water will replenish your body with everything you need after a workout. If you need a little more calcium, blend in some juiced spinach. If you need protein on the fly, juice some kale and mix it into the drink.

If you need a quick boost of energy, juice two carrots, one orange, and some strawberries. This is a quick pick-me-up when your energy levels are plummeting.

Don't throw away the pulp...

There are lots of uses for the pulp left over from juicing. You can mix them with chia seeds and water, making a paste and then dehydrate them for delicious crackers that you can use for homemade dips or put hummus spread on them for a healthy snack. Don't like hummus? Make your favorite dips with unsweetened Greek yogurt. To tame the bitter taste of the yogurt you can add just a touch of sea salt and Grade A Maple syrup.

If you need something sweet, melt unsweetened cacao bars, Grade A maple syrup, and coconut flakes for a healthy taste of something sweet without having to reach for a candy bar. Add a nut butter to make it protein-packed.

On days that you don't feel like cooking, make meals and snacks ahead of time to plan for those days. If you are making trail mixes, make enough for a week or two and store it in an air-tight container. Buy meats for more than one meal, marinate them, and store them in the freezer for a quick meal.

A few final words...

Don't get discouraged. It will take about three weeks to start seeing a difference. Your body has to detox before it rebuilds and heals itself. In the meantime, keep following the diet. It will take six weeks to start getting back to your former self, and by that time, you'll be used to your new lifestyle and wonder how you ever lived like you did before you started to reset your adrenals.

You will go through withdrawals. Your body will crave the sugar and caffeine you left behind. It will take 21 days for your body to stop with the symptoms of withdrawal, which includes cravings.

Look online for advice and support. You are not alone with your illness. There are others out there that have gone through what you are, and have made it back to leading a healthy and productive life. They will be more than willing to help you feel better.

Listen to your body. Everyone's body is different and will respond to a new lifestyle differently. Keep a diary, whether written or verbal. This will help you pinpoint the foods your body reacts to negatively or favorably. It is a process, but one that will be worth it in the end.

Your new lifestyle will be little more costly than the last. Keep an eye out for sales, coupons and deals to help you save money while getting your health back.

Commit to trying one new food each week that is on your list of foods to eat. This will broaden your menu, and you may be surprised as to what you will like. Try different way to prepare foods that you did not like before. You may find out that you didn't like it just because of the way it was prepared. If you've only had green beans out of a can, try fresh and sauté them with a little bacon grease and roasted garlic and almond slivers.

Use broths to cook with

Take a carcass, like a chicken carcass; place it in a pot with carrots, celery, onion, garlic and your choice of seasonings. Cover all of it with water. Bring it to a boil, and then allow it to simmer, with the lid on it until all the meat has fallen off the bones.

The bones contain marrow which is also good for resetting adrenals. Now, you have a healthy broth you can use to cook rice, soups, and other grains, like quinoa. You can also use broths to make sauces and gravies.

Avoid stressful situations when possible. When it isn't possible, learn to take in stride, not letting the situation get to you. When you feel you are holding back or about to lose your temper, go for a walk or take a deep breath and walk away from the situation. This may take practice and time, but in the long run, you'll feel better and be a better person over-all.

The main thing is to remember that you are doing this for you. Only you can take care of your body the way it needs to be cared for and maintained. Once you start on the path to resetting your adrenals, don't stop or give up. Your health is at stake. Isn't that reason enough?

Resources:

Tenney, Louise, MH. Today's Herbal Health, 6th ed.
http://drhyman.com/blog/2013/09/17/push-pause-button-adrenal-burnout/
http://empoweredsustenance.com/adaptogenic-sports-drink/
https://blissreturned.wordpress.com/2012/02/05/fruits-and-vegetable-list-of-low-and-high-sugar-fruit-and-vegetable/
http://amazingwellnessmag.com/the-adrenal-reset-diet/